*May you be inspired to
stand strong against life's challenges*

Words
for the Cure

*Inspiration, Hope, and Comfort
for Today and Tomorrow*

Presented by
SUSAN G.
KOMEN
FOR THE
CURE

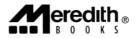

Meredith Books
1716 Locust Street
Des Moines, Iowa 50309–3023
meredithbooks.com

Printed in China.

First Edition.
Library of Congress Control Number: 2007925127
ISBN: 978-0-696-23812-3

ABOUT THIS BOOK *A diagnosis of breast cancer brings with it a wide range of emotions that often include shock, fear, denial, sadness, and anger. And although time may lessen the intensity of such feelings, it likely won't wash them away completely. Studies show that support from a variety of formal and informal sources can have real quality-of-life benefits, including improvements in mood, ability to cope, and reduced levels of stress. We offer this book as one of those sources.*

Each quote contained in this book is a thought shared in a moment in time by someone touched by breast cancer. These quotes are taken from a variety of sources: newspaper or magazine interviews, public speeches, books, or websites. As you open to any page, you will find insights into your own thoughts and emotions. And you can know that you are not alone. We invite you to find inspiration in the strength of these others who have faced their own personal struggles with the disease.

Dear Friends,

Thank you for picking up this copy of Words for the Cure. Whether you are dealing with a life-threatening illness yourself or sharing the journey with someone who is, you will visit these pages again and again, taking with you something new, thought provoking, and life affirming each time.

As a breast cancer survivor, I remember the importance of kind words, encouragement, hope, and inspiration when my diagnosis and treatment left me feeling overwhelmed with fear and confusion. Life-threatening illness can alter your view of yourself and your ability to cope. When serious illness becomes your new reality, it's important to pause, to draw close to friends, and to know that you are not alone.

The words and images in this book are like footprints on a beach left by friends on a similar journey all leading you to a place of quiet reflection and peace.

When the Meredith Corporation unveiled its plans to produce Words for the Cure, I enthusiastically supported it on behalf of Susan G. Komen for the Cure, the organization

I founded 25 years ago to honor my beloved big sister, Susan G. Komen, who died of breast cancer at age 36. She was my hero and my best friend. She brought light to those around her. I miss her every day, but that light still shines, guiding me and Komen for the Cure in its quest to end breast cancer forever.

Words for the Cure speaks volumes about hope, about determination, and about the resilience of the human spirit in the face of fear.

A good book can, indeed, be a very good friend. This is a friend you'll turn to time and time again.

Sincerely,

Nancy G. Brinker

Nancy Goodman Brinker
Founder, Susan G. Komen
for the Cure

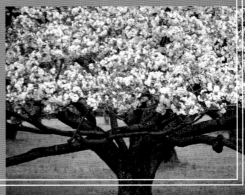

66 My promise and Susan G. Komen for the Cure's promise is this: to save lives and end breast cancer forever by empowering people, ensuring quality care for all, and energizing science to find the cures. 99

–HALA MODDELMOG

As a 5-year breast cancer survivor and former Fortune 500 executive, Hala Moddelmog joined the Susan G. Komen Foundation as CEO to work to eradicate breast cancer.

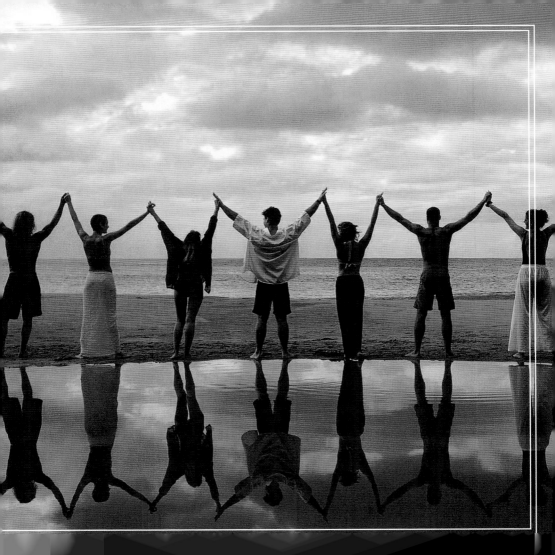

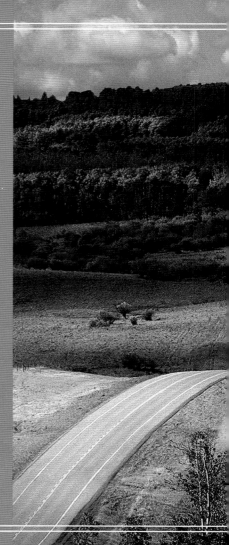

> **"I don't know what my path is yet. I'm just walking on it."**
> **–OLIVIA NEWTON-JOHN**

Best known for her role as Sandy in *Grease*, Olivia Newton-John discovered and successfully battled breast cancer in 1992.

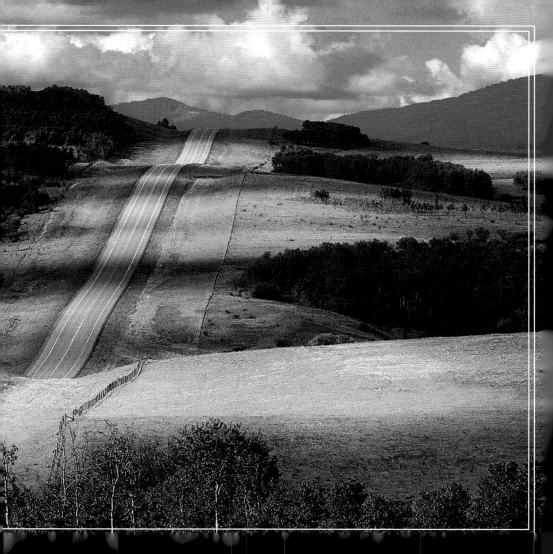

> **"When I got the news, I was shocked. I thought, 'I couldn't possibly have breast cancer. Men don't get this.' Whether it's breast cancer or heart disease, [men need to] start taking their health more seriously."**
>
> **—RICHARD ROUNDTREE**

While the occurrence of breast cancer in men is much lower, the death rate is significantly higher. Actor Richard Roundtree attributes his successful fight to heading straight to a doctor when he felt a lump.

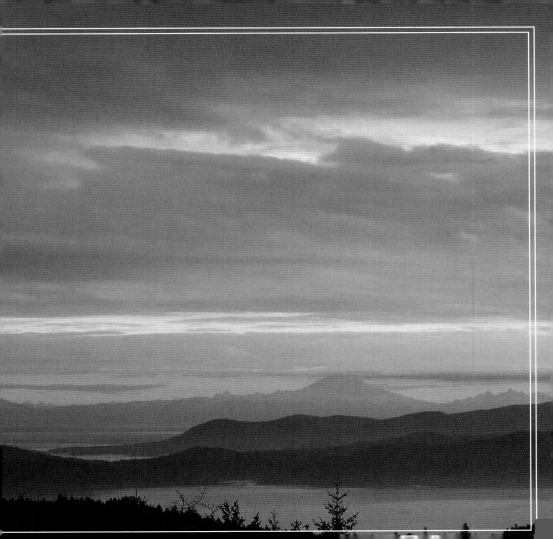

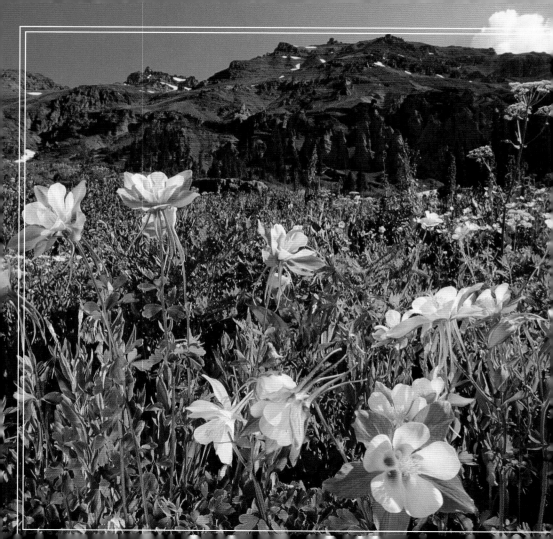

❝ *People are always telling me that change is good. But all that means is that something you didn't want to happen has happened.* **❞**

—MEG RYAN

Susan Ryan Jordan, mother of actress Meg Ryan, published a book entitled *The Immune Spirit* about her struggle with breast cancer and the difficulty it caused in her relationship with her daughter. Meg Ryan's character shared this thought in *You've Got Mail*.

66 *When a woman is faced with breast cancer and has to deal with the physical and emotional changes it brings, she must remember that no matter what those changes are, she is still beautiful inside and out, and that her heart, spirit, and faith will help her to fight and overcome the disease.* 99

–PATTI LABELLE

Having lost three sisters and her mother to various forms of cancer, singer, actress, and advocate Patti LaBelle works to spread the word about the disease.

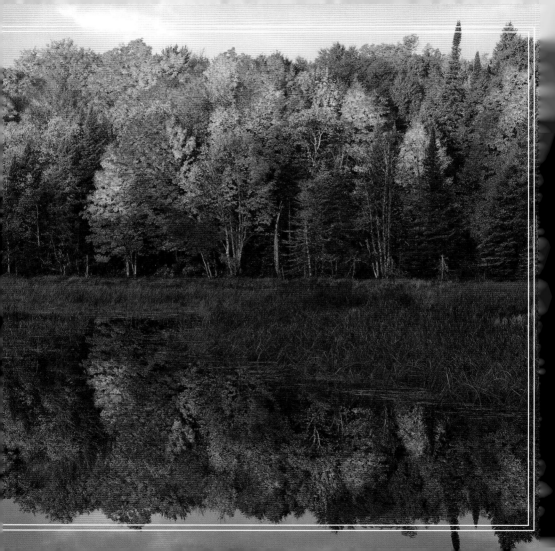

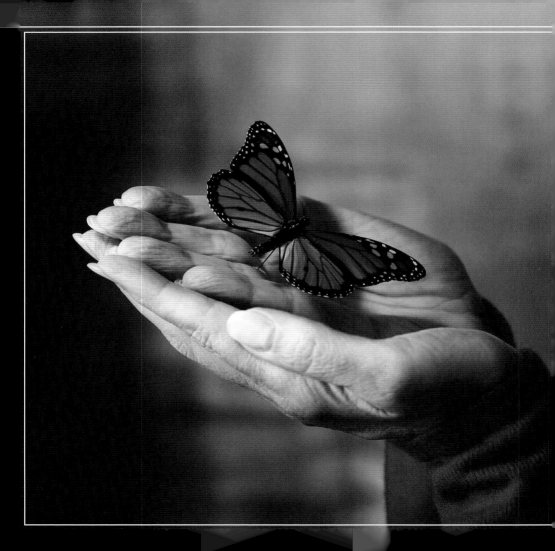

❝ *This diagnosis is a reminder that this is the life you've got. And you're not getting another one. Whatever has happened, you have to take this life and treasure and protect it.* **❞**

—ELIZABETH EDWARDS

Elizabeth Edwards, lawyer and wife of former North Carolina senator John Edwards, noticed a large lump in her breast just two weeks before the 2004 presidential election. She shared this thought and others on the *Today* show and in a book that followed.

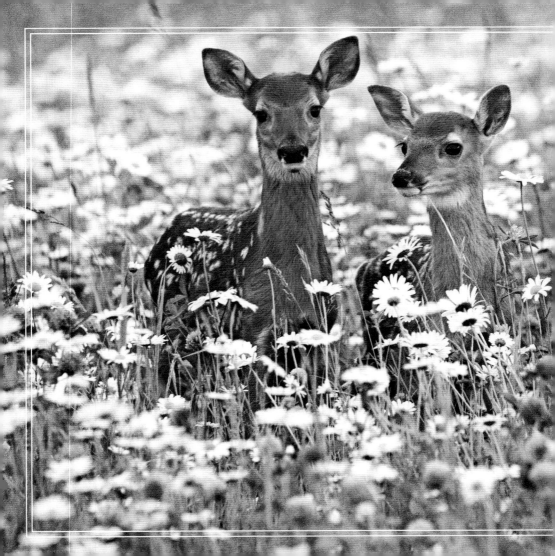

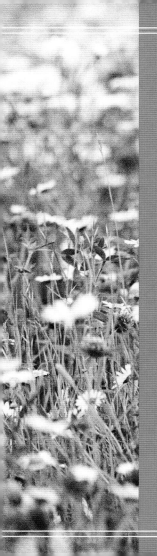

> **" Women need to know what their options are. Some are afraid they are dying, and that's not necessarily [going to happen]. The earlier you find [breast cancer], the better your chances of survival."**

–DIAHANN CARROLL

Actress and survivor Diahann Carroll's breast cancer was less than a centimeter in size when it was detected and completely removed by a lumpectomy. She shared this thought in *Ebony* magazine.

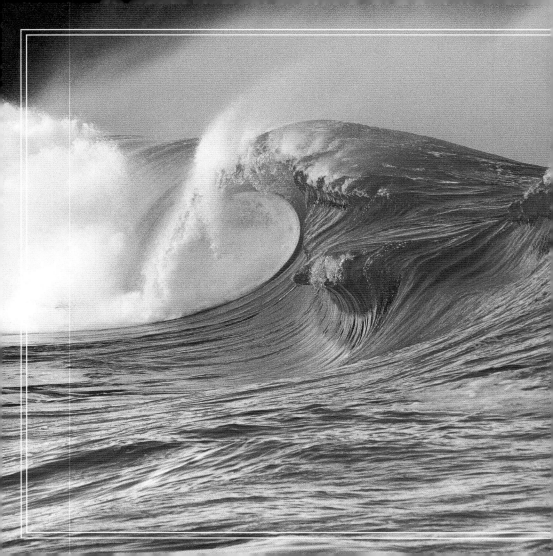

> **"It's how you handle adversity, not how it affects you. The main thing is never quit, never quit, never quit."**
>
> **—BILL CLINTON**

Former President of the United States Bill Clinton lost his mother, Virginia, to breast cancer in 1994.

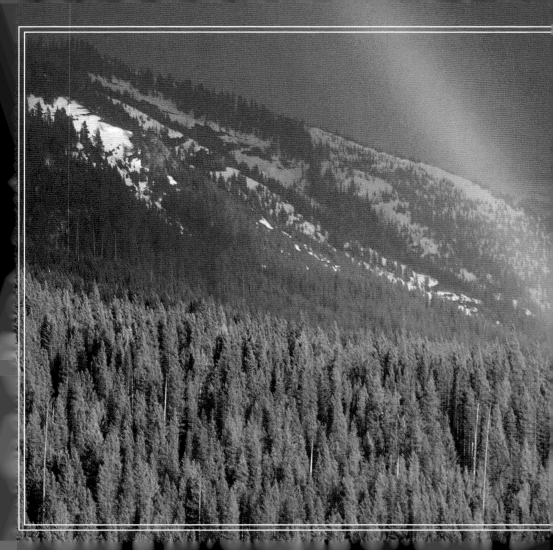

**66** You're never guaranteed about next year. People ask what you think of next season; you have to seize the opportunities when they're in front of you. **99**

—BRETT FAVRE

NFL quarterback Brett Favre supported his wife through her struggle with breast cancer in 2004 and continues to support the cause.

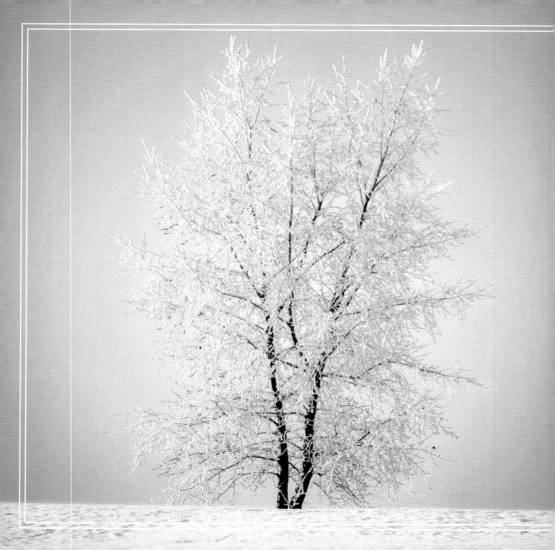

> **❝** *I think it's important that we don't all have to hold our heads high all the time saying everything's fine.* **❞**
> **—NICOLE KIDMAN**

At age 17 actress Nicole Kidman stopped working for two years to learn massage so that she could provide physical therapy to her mother (her mom eventually beat the breast cancer). Kidman's parents moved to the U.S. to allow her biochemist father to pursue his research on breast cancer.

> **"I didn't want to live my life as a victim; I didn't want to use the excuse that I coulda or shoulda or woulda had a great life but I had some bad luck. It has always been the 'bad luck' or the negatives in my life that have taught me and shaped me, and I wasn't going to lose this time around. Cancer was going to be my blessing. I was going to learn and grow and survive my way."**
>
> **—SUZANNE SOMERS**

Actress, author, and survivor Suzanne Somers wrote this thought in her book *The Sexy Years*.

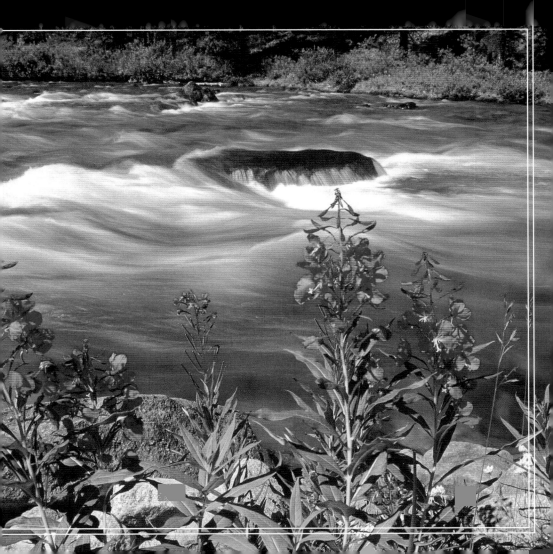

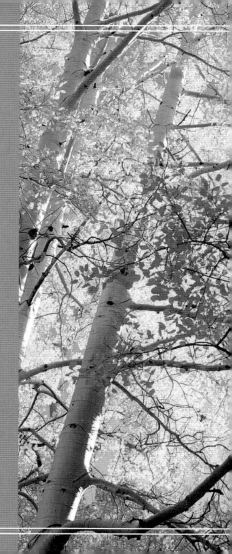

> **"** *Life presents you with choices that you then have to deal with and adapt to.* **"**
>
> **–COKIE ROBERTS**

Cokie Roberts made these remarks to the 1994 graduating class of Wellesley College. This political journalist was diagnosed at age 58 when a small tumor was discovered in her left breast. She underwent surgery and recovered.

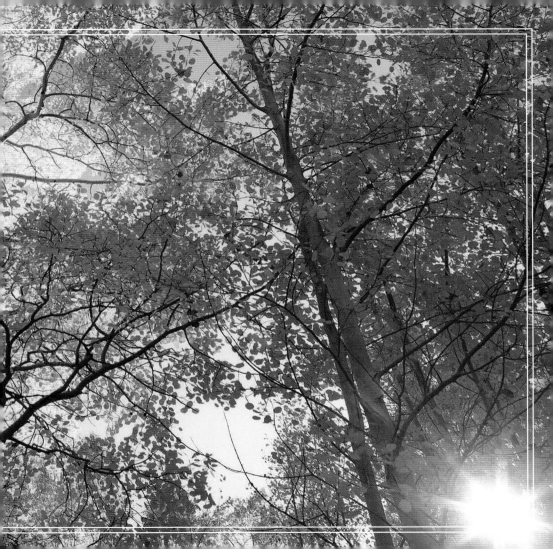

> *Believe in who you are, believe in what you feel, your power will come from that.*
>
> **—MELISSA ETHERIDGE**

Academy Award-winning musician Melissa Etheridge discovered a lump in her breast in 2004 at age 43. After surgery, chemo, and radiation, she was cancer-free.

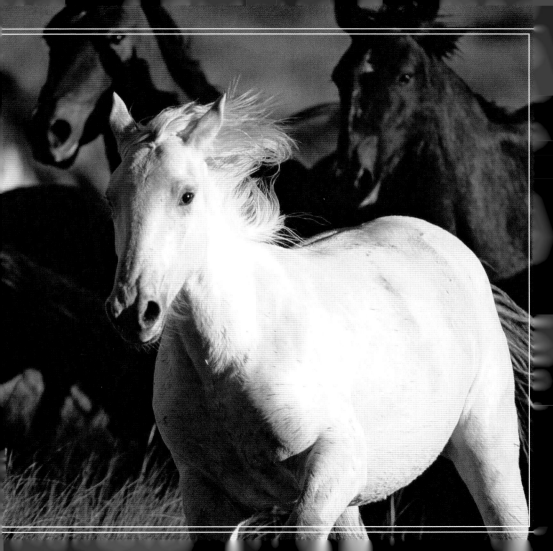

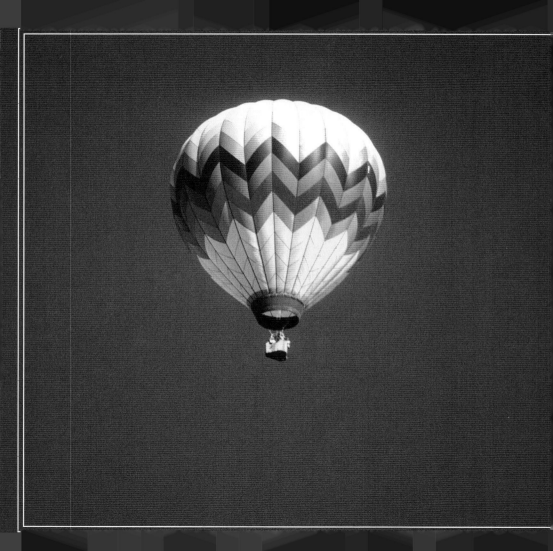

"Without leaps of imagination, or dreaming, we lose the excitement of possibilities. Dreaming, after all, is a form of planning."

—GLORIA STEINEM

Best known as a supporter of the women's movement, Gloria Steinem was stricken with breast cancer in 1986.

> **❝** Now is the accepted time, not tomorrow, not some more convenient season. It is today that our best work can be done and not some future day or future year. It is today that we fit ourselves for the greater usefulness of tomorrow. Today is the seed time, now are the hours of work, and tomorrow comes the harvest and the playtime. **❞**

—W.E.B. DU BOIS

The wife of African-American writer and thinker W.E.B. Du Bois lost her battle with breast cancer in 1977.

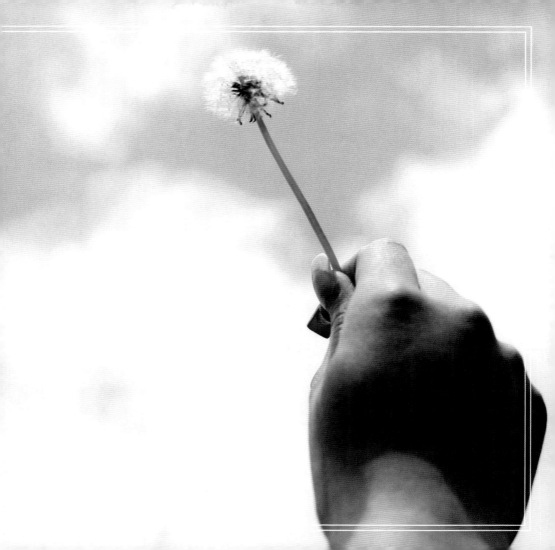

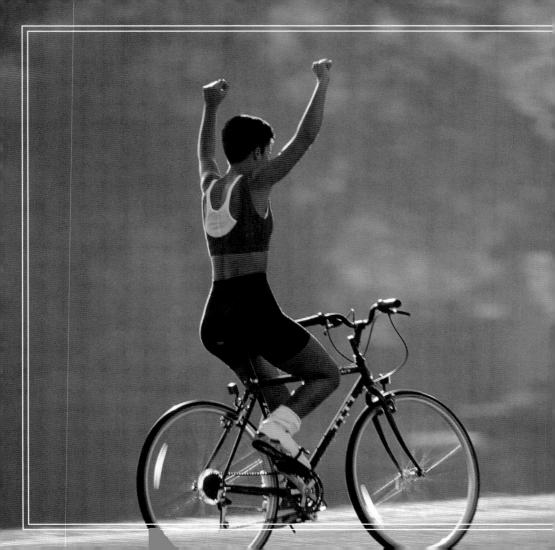

&6&6 *If children have the ability to ignore all odds and percentages, then maybe we can all learn from them. When you think about it, what other choice is there but to hope? We have two options, medically and emotionally: Give up, or fight like hell.* **99**

—LANCE ARMSTRONG

No stranger to cancer himself, Lance Armstrong was able to share his perspective when then-fiancée Sheryl Crow was diagnosed with breast cancer.

> **The key to life is accepting challenges. Once someone stops doing this, he's dead.**
>
> —BETTE DAVIS

This first lady of the American screen lost her battle with breast cancer in 1989.

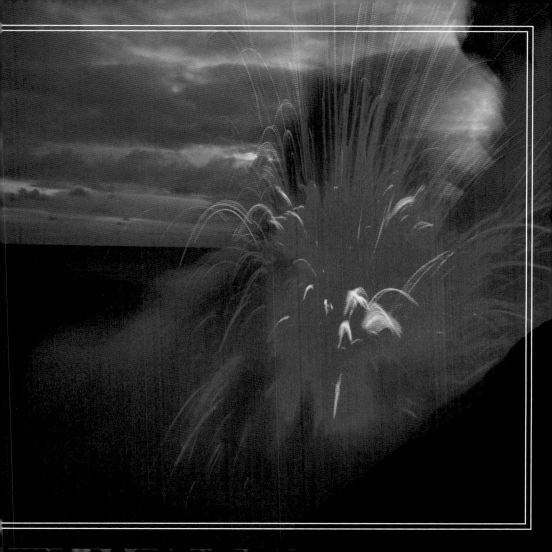

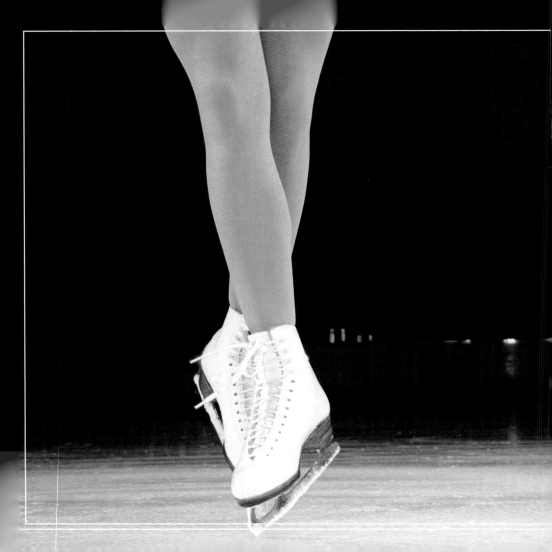

When the going got tough, I really had to draw on many of the same competitive instincts I did when I was skating. I really had to put my head down and stay positive. I had to fight.

—PEGGY FLEMING

Peggy Fleming made this statement in a newspaper interview after the figure skater found a lump in her breast in 1998. The cancer was detected in its early stages and surgery was successful.

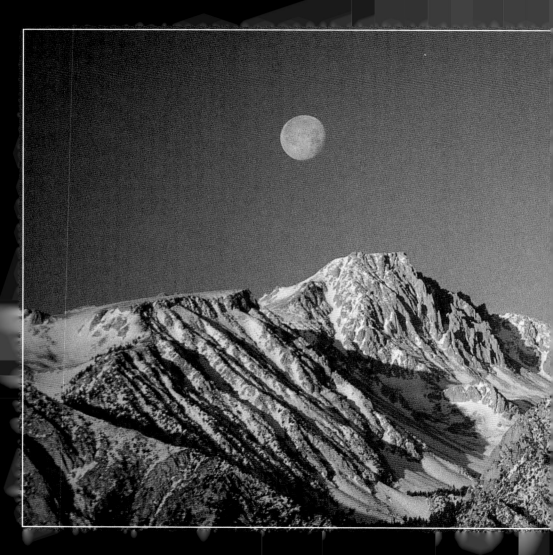

❝ I've been motivated by overcoming challenge and overcoming the hurdles and obstacles that face me. There still is plenty out there to get motivated by. ❞

—ANDRE AGASSI

Tennis pro Andre Agassi chose to take two months off from the game after he learned that his mother and sister were both diagnosed with breast cancer in 2000.

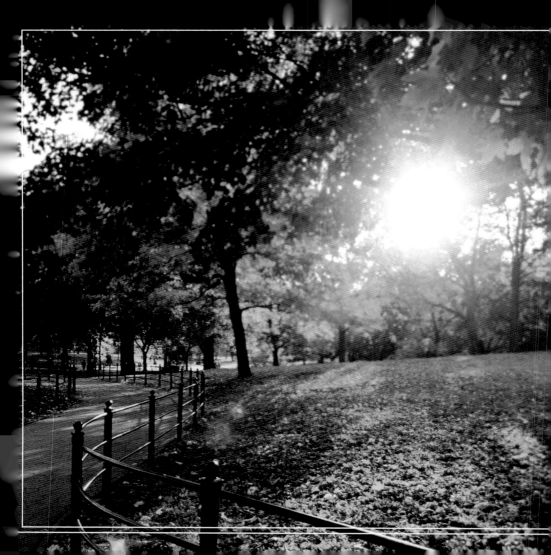

> **" Take the back roads instead of the highways. "**
>
> **–MINNIE PEARL**

After surviving breast cancer through aggressive treatments including a double mastectomy and radiation therapy, this comedian became a spokeswoman for the medical center in Nashville where she had been treated.

> **" The work of today is the history of tomorrow, and we are its makers. "**
> **–JULIETTE GORDON LOW**

Founder of the Girls Scouts of the USA, Juliette Gordon Low discovered her breast cancer in 1923 and lost her life to it in 1927.

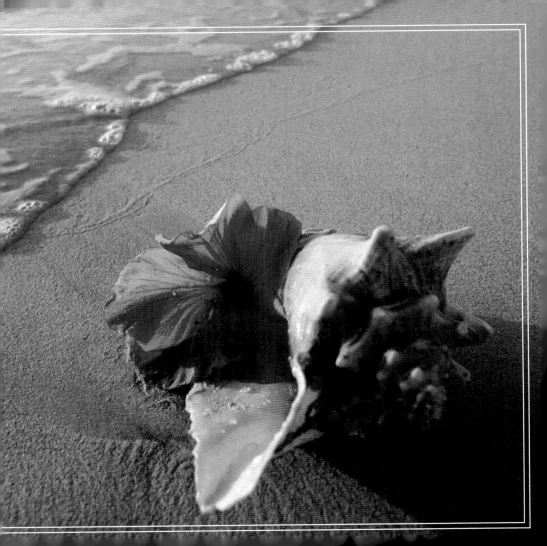

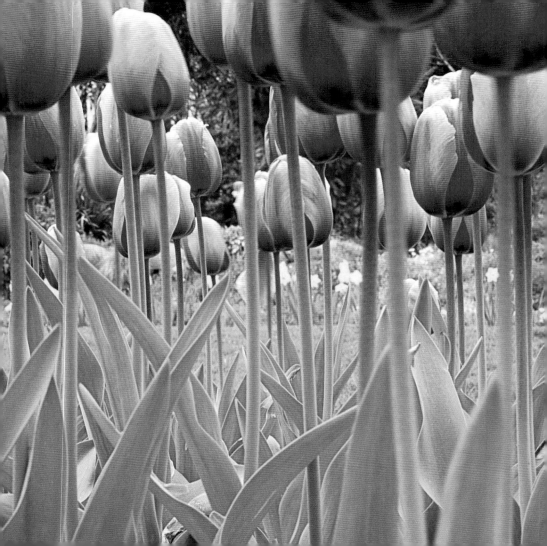

❝ *Do the best you can in every task, no matter how unimportant it may seem at the time. No one learns more about a problem than the person at the bottom.* **❞**

—SANDRA DAY O'CONNOR

This first woman appointed to the U.S. Supreme Court, Sandra Day O'Connor returned to the bench just 10 days after her mastectomy in 1988.

> **"I am a big believer that eventually everything comes back to you. You get back what you give out."**
>
> —NANCY REAGAN

Former First Lady Nancy Reagan made the controversial choice for a modified radical mastectomy for her breast cancer detected in 1987.

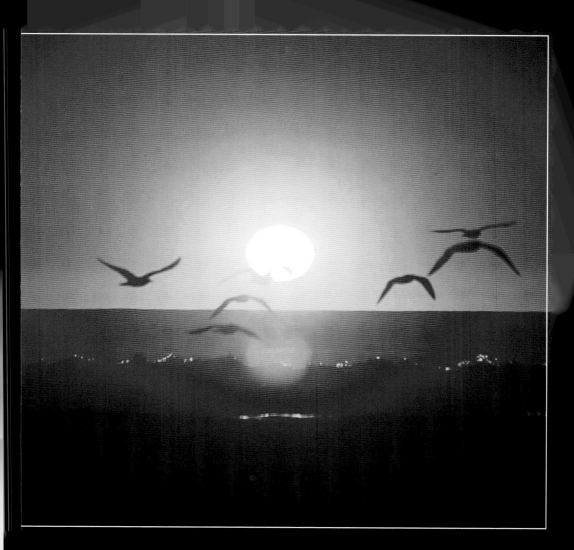

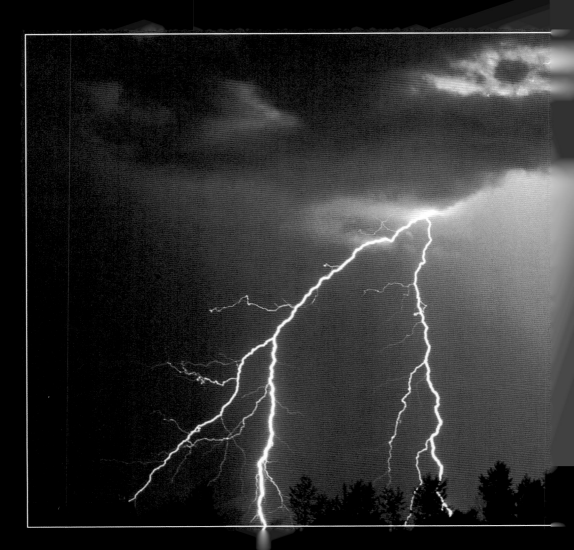

> **❝** *We don't know what's going to happen in the next moment. Enjoy all the tiny details, and appreciate what you have.* **❞**
> **—BRITTANY MURPHY**

Sharon Murphy, Brittany's mom, has faced breast cancer twice and had a double mastectomy. The actress is also relieved about her own health: In 2006 she found two lumps in her right breast, which, happily, turned out to be benign.

❝ *Breast cancer strikes a cultural bone with me. Many in the Latino community avoid discussing this topic. I hope that hearing from me, a Latino man who lost his mother to breast cancer, will encourage others to take care of the women in their lives.* **❞**

–RICARDO CHAVIRA

Desperate Housewives actor and advocate Ricardo Chavira was only 15 when he lost his mother..

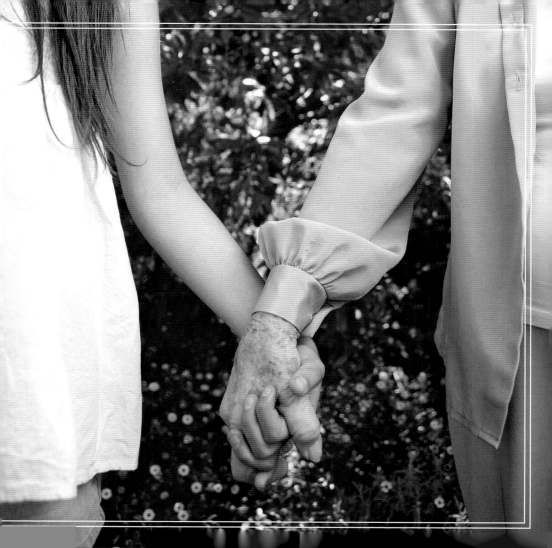

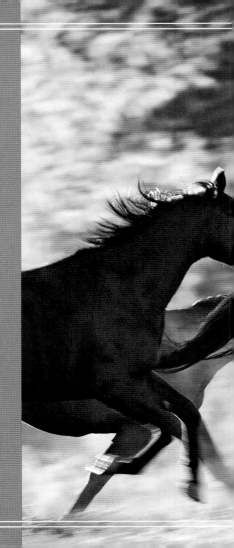

"*I don't know any other way to lead but by example.*"

–DON SHULA

Former coach of the Miami Dolphins Don Shula created the Don Shula Foundation for breast cancer research after losing his wife to the disease in 1991.

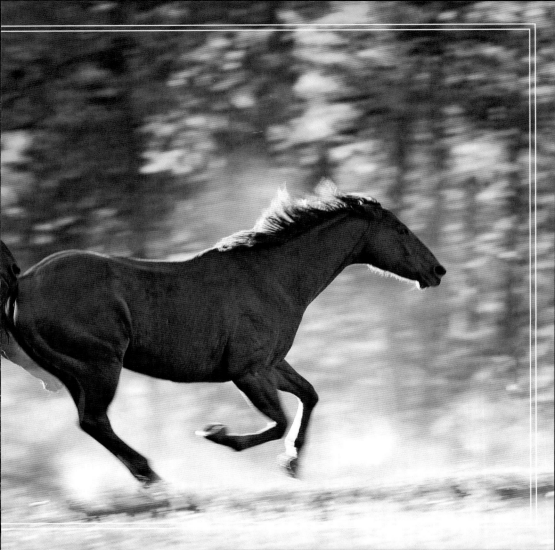

66 *I love that kind of thought: All the information for a tree was in an acorn—the tree was somehow in there.* **99**
–PAUL McCARTNEY

This former Beatle lost his wife Linda to breast cancer.

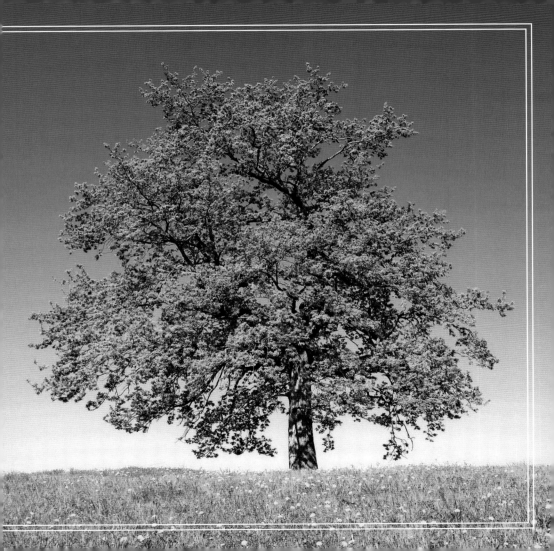

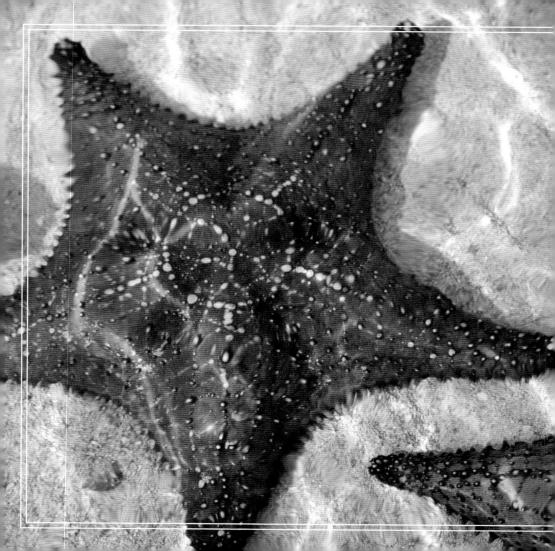

> **66** *I never felt a psychic wound; I never felt hopelessly mutilated. After all, Jerry and I had been married a good many years, and our love had proved itself. I had no reason to doubt my husband. If he'd lost a leg, I wouldn't have deserted him, and I knew he wouldn't desert me because I was unfortunate enough to have had a mastectomy.* **99**

—BETTY FORD

This former First Lady publicly shared her diagnosis and mastectomy at a time when the topic was still taboo. Within weeks thousands of women who had been reluctant to examine their breasts inundated cancer screening centers.

❝ To be brave is to love someone unconditionally, without expecting anything in return. To just give. That takes courage, because we don't want to fall on our faces or leave ourselves open to hurt.❞

—MADONNA

This singer lost her mother to breast cancer as a young child.

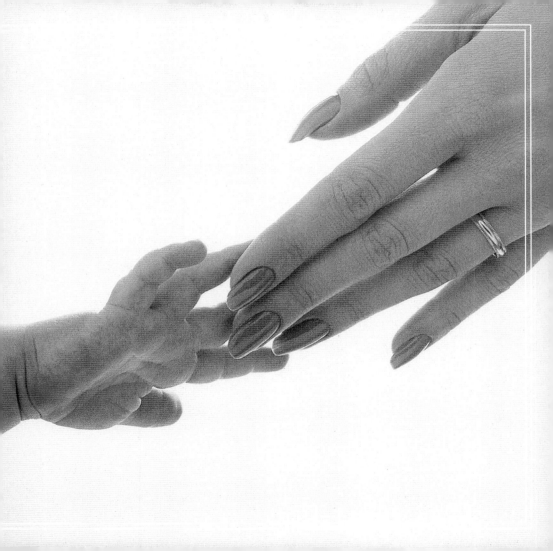

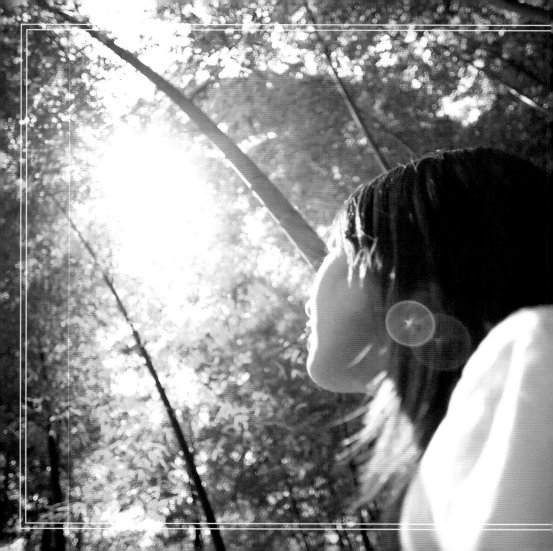

> **❝** I was seventeen when my mother passed away . . . I was heartbroken. Nothing mattered to me anymore. I thought seriously about not finishing high school, even of dropping out of boxing. Not one day passes that I don't think about my mother. And to be honest, there are still times when it's a lonely world without her. But I feel that I was blessed to have her in my life, and I believe she's still looking out for me. **❞**

—OSCAR DE LA HOYA

This pro boxer's mom lost her life to breast cancer at the age of 38. Her memory inspired him to go on to win an Olympic gold medal.

> **"** *Angels are like diamonds. They can't be made, you have to find them. Each one is unique.* **"**
> —JACLYN SMITH

This former Charlie's Angel discovered a lump during a routine checkup in 2002 and underwent a lumpectomy and radiation therapy the following month. Her character shared this thought in a cameo appearance in *Charlie's Angels: Full Throttle*.

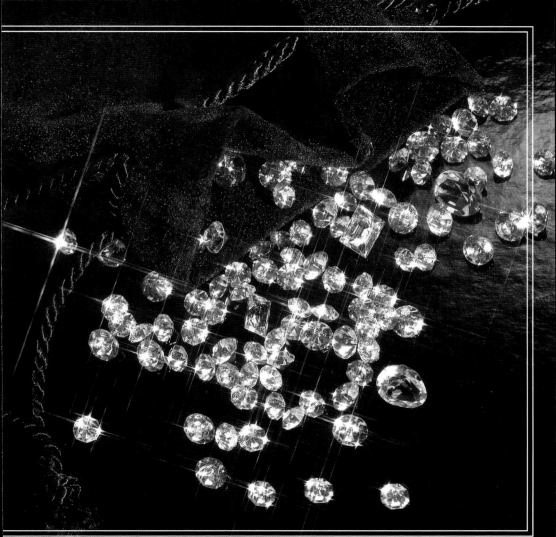

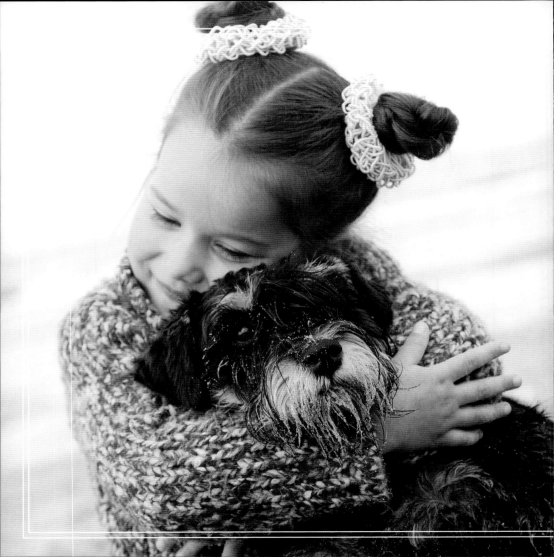

> **❝** *Compassion is the foundation of everything positive, everything good. If you carry the power of compassion to the marketplace and the dinner table, you can make your life really count.* **❞**
> —RUE McCLANAHAN

This Emmy-winning actress was diagnosed with breast cancer on the day that her soon-to-be fiancé first told her that he loved her.

❝ Many of us at Pole are searchers, many are travelers, and many have come, as I did, to destroy demons and to find answers . . . we have found and conquered demons, thoughts, weaknesses, questioning of the self, that we did not before know existed. And in doing so, we have learned that those things that plagued us in the world were not important or had gone to rest years ago. ❞

—DR. JERRI NIELSEN

Dr. Nielsen was 46 when she took a job as the only doctor on a South Pole station. Only a week into the no-travel portion of winter, she discovered her accelerated breast cancer and was forced to self-treat.

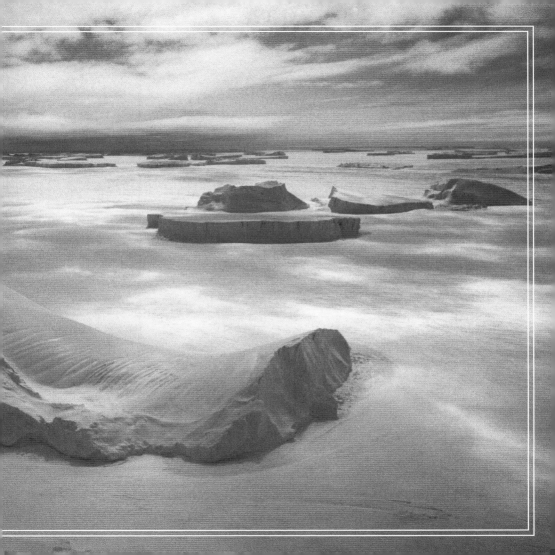

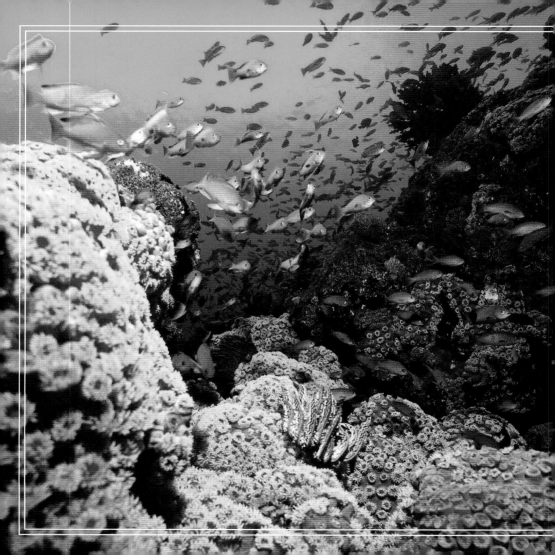

> **❝On chemotherapy:**
> *I lost everything—my hair, my eyebrows, eyelashes—and yet I still had to shave my legs. The one place a woman really wants to lose hair, and I didn't.❞*
>
> —**DEANNA FAVRE**

Deanna Favre, wife of NFL superstar Brett Favre, created The Deanna Favre Hope Foundation after her diagnosis in 2004. It supports breast cancer education and women's breast imaging and diagnosis services for all women, including those who are medically underserved.

66 I have had a wonderful life. I have never regretted what I did. I regret things I didn't do. All my life I've done things at a moment's notice. Those are the things I remember. I was given courage, a sense of adventure, and a little bit of humor. 99

—INGRID BERGMAN

Swedish-born actress Ingrid Bergman, winner of three Academy Awards, succumbed to complications of breast cancer on her birthday in 1982.

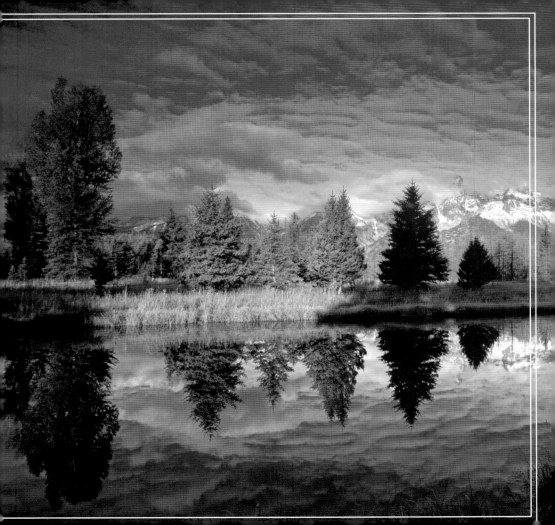

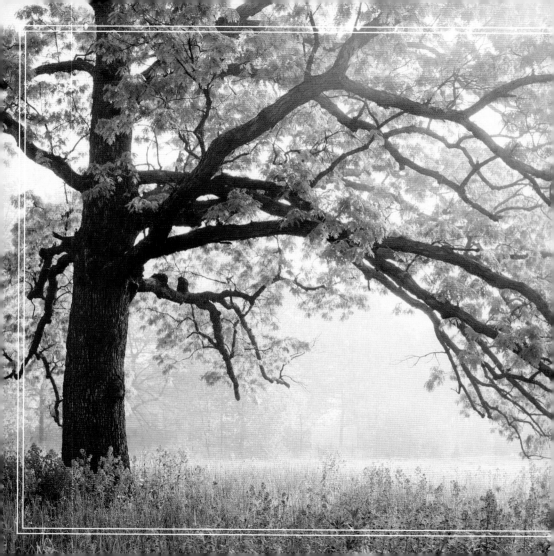

" *I took a topless photo for* SELF *magazine after my mastectomy to show other young women what a mastectomy with reconstruction looked like. I thought that I was posing to inspire another woman (and nearly chickened out) but somehow that photo made me see a 'me' I had never seen . . . it was the first time I ever thought I looked beautiful . . . ever.* **"**

—GERALYN LUCAS

Journalist Geralyn Lucas discovered her
cancer at age 27 and wrote a book entitled
Why I Wore Lipstick to My Mastectomy.

66 *But when this happens to you—and I think other people would identify with this—suddenly, colors are brighter. You see everything.* **99**

–LYNN REDGRAVE

Actress Lynn Redgrave
suffered through, worked through,
and, most important, lived through
her battle with breast cancer.

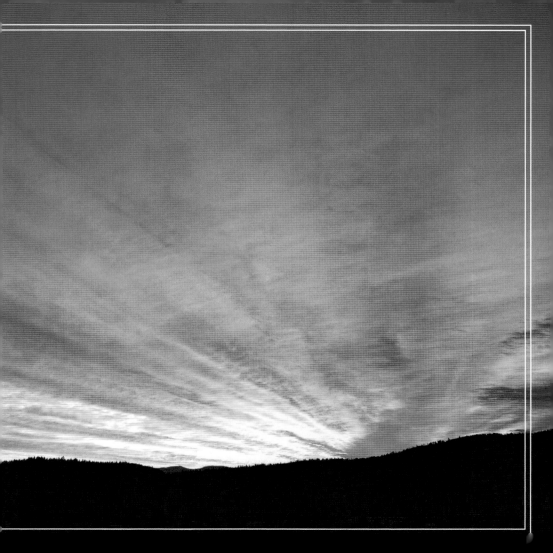

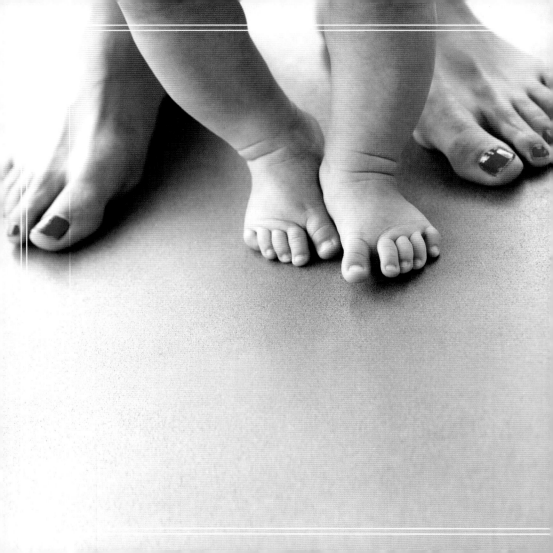

> **"I want to live, I want to get married, I want to have children, and I want to continue working. I will not give up."**
>
> —ADAMARI LÓPEZ

Latina actress Adamari López
announced her breast cancer
diagnosis in 2005 at the age of 34.

" *The only positive thing you can really gain through losing someone is learning and teaching other people. So I hope to teach other people, and I hope to learn.* **"**

—STELLA McCARTNEY

Fashion designer and advocate
Stella McCartney lost her mother,
Linda McCartney, to breast cancer and
shared this thought in an interview
on the U.K.'s Sky Television.

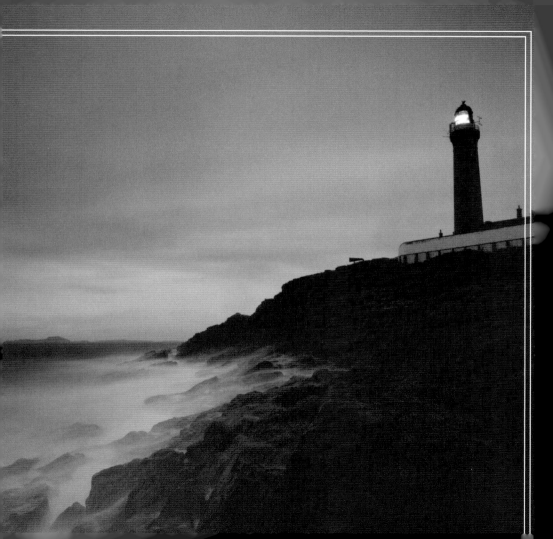

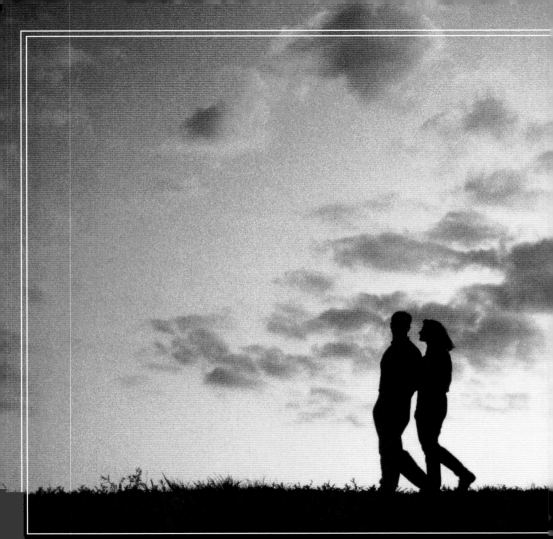

> **"** *The last 20 years have been remarkable for me and my husband, Mike. We've learned to value each other in a new way, and our love has gotten deeper every year. Mike says it's because we now realize that we are going to die. Maybe not from breast cancer but from something. And so the question becomes, 'How do we want to live?'* **"**

—JILL EIKENBERRY

Best known for her work on *L.A. Law*, Jill Eikenberry was performing her first breast self-exam and felt a lump. Her doctor confirmed breast cancer and recommended a mastectomy, but she sought a second opinion. Lumpectomy and radiation therapies were recommended, and her breast was saved.

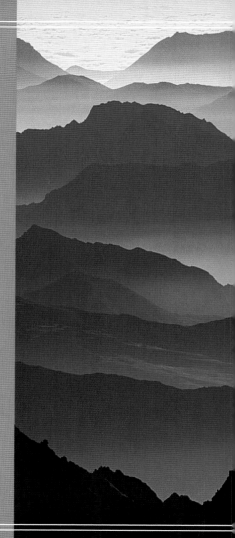

❝*I feel more inspired than ever, and think that I will finally achieve what I have long been wishing for: a balance of work and privacy—a harmony.***❞**

–KYLIE MINOGUE

This Australian pop star postponed her tour when diagnosed with breast cancer in 2005.

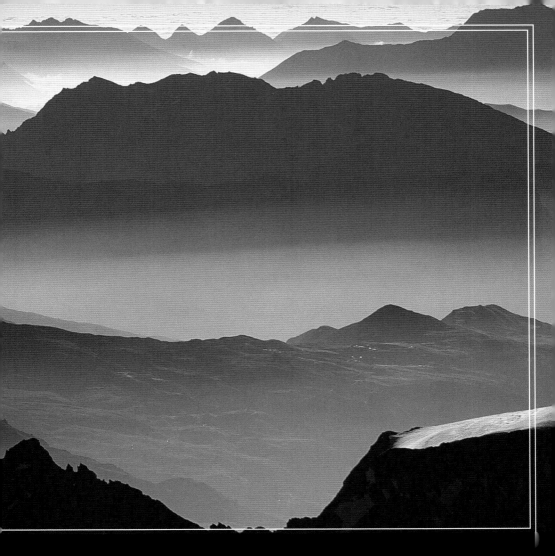

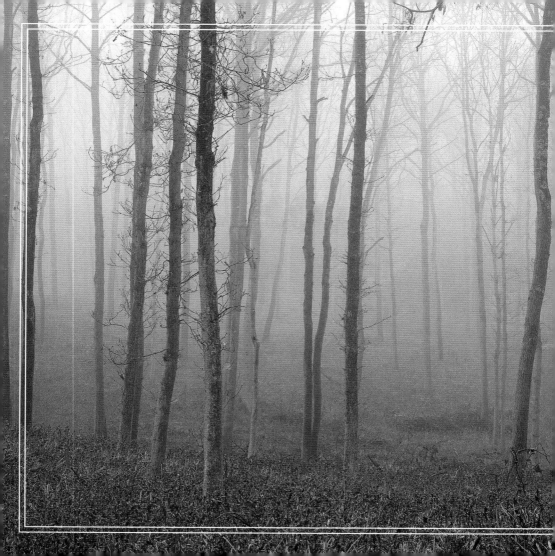

> **"I feel keenly aware of how precious and fleeting life is, and I hope I will never forget what the experience has taught me . . . who I am, who I want to be, who I can never be again. It was a hard time, but I'd rather have the really hard stuff than to never know what I know now."**
>
> **—SHERYL CROW**

Singer and survivor Sheryl Crow
shared this thought on her website,
sherylcrow.com.

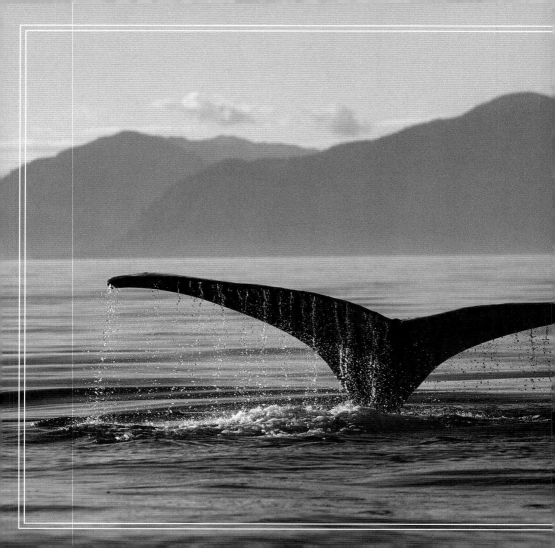

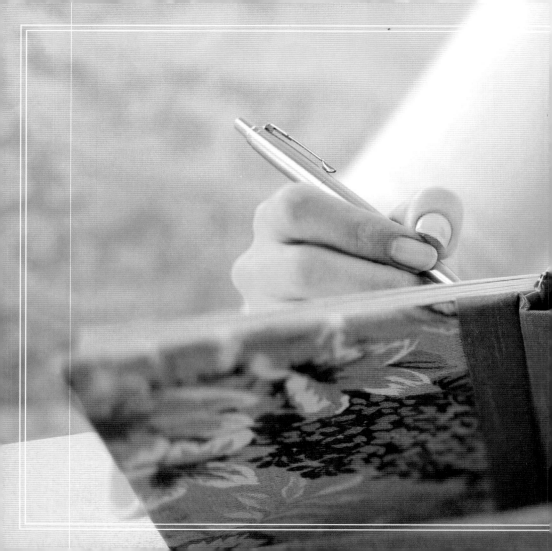

> **" When I stand before God at the end of my life, I would hope that I would not have a single bit of talent left and could say, 'I used everything you gave me.' "**
>
> **—ERMA BOMBECK**

Humor columnist Erma Bombeck was diagnosed with breast cancer and underwent a mastectomy in 1992.

> **" A really strong woman accepts the war she went through and is ennobled by her scars. "**
>
> **–CARLY SIMON**

Carly Simon underwent a mastectomy and reconstructive surgery for breast cancer in 1997 and was able to sing about it on her album *The Bedroom Tapes*.

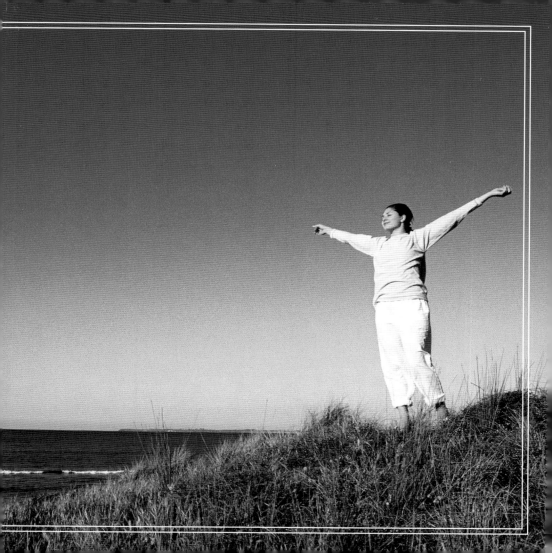

What Kind of Promise Will You Make?

Susan G. Komen for the Cure was born in a special promise made between two sisters. More than 25 years ago, Nancy G. Brinker promised her dying sister, Susan G. Komen, she would do everything in her power to end breast cancer forever. That promise became Susan G. Komen for the Cure and launched the global breast cancer movement.

Want to make the Susan G. Komen for the Cure promise your own?

The organization has ways for everyone to join the fight to end breast cancer forever. Find a way that moves you.

Any number of opportunities are at your fingertips when you visit Komen for the Cure's awardwinning website, www.komen.org. Here you can read about the organization, find out about the latest breast cancer advancements, and the phenomenal work of Komen Affiliates across the United States and in three foreign countries.

- Click on *Affiliates* and learn how to become a breast cancer activist by teaming up with your local Komen Affiliate.
- Find a Susan G. Komen Race for the Cure® or a Breast Cancer 3-Day event in a community near you and start training today. Or volunteer to support the Komen Race for the Cure Series® and its 1.6 million annual participants!
- Click on *Public Policy* and read up on the issues. Sign up for Komen's activist-powered eChampions online advocacy program. Let your voice and opinions be heard by your local, state, and federal legislators about important breast cancer issues.
- Click on *Donations* and choose a way that makes sense for you to support Komen's important work.
- Like to shop? Want to do it for a good cause? Visit *Marketplace* and find great merchandise with a pink ribbon theme and a purpose—helping to end breast cancer forever.
- Or click on *Partners* and find out what everyday products (and some very special ones) Komen partners have created as part of their own promise to get active in the fight against breast cancer.

Thank you for helping Susan G. Komen for the Cure keep its promise to save lives, deliver the cures, and end breast cancer forever.